I0422686

Printed September 2017

DISCLAIMER

The information in this book is for general education. So, if you have any health issues, I strongly advise that you work with your health care practitioner to use this information in the best possible way to promote your health and wellbeing.

DEDICATION

I dedicate this book to God Almighty who gave me the wisdom and strength to put the book together.

WHAT!!! AFRICAN FOOD! HEALTHY LIFESTYLE? YOU'VE GOT TO BE KIDDING ME!

Table of Contents

INTORDUCTION 6

YOU ARE WHAT YOU EAT............................6

MY TESTIMONY 8

GLYCEMIC INDEX/ GLYCEMIC LOAD; WHAT ARE THEY?...9

HIGH GLYCEMIC 10

LOW GLYCEMIC INDEX.............................10

HIGH GLYCEMIC AND LOW GLYCEMIC INDEX 11

GLYCEMIC LOAD 13

WHAT IS GLYCEMIC LOAD? 13

CAUTION..15

CHAPTER 2 16

WHAT I DID DO FOR THE SEVEN WEEKS 16

POST SEVEN WEEKS – LIFESTYLE.........................18

CHAPTER 3 24

SPECIFIC FOOD RECOMMENDATION 24

SNACKING HABIT WILL NOT SUFFER 28

WHY I HAD TO STOP THE WHEAT PRODUCTS ...28

CHAPTER 4 31

WHY I CHOSE SOME OF THE LOW GLYCEMIC INDEX FOOD I EAT NOW.............................31

BENEFITS OF YAMS 31

BENEFITS OF OATMEAL.............................33

BENEFITS OF QUINOA 33

BENEFITS OF RYE 34

BENEFITS OF BUCKWHEAT 34

CHAPTER 5 35

GENERAL RECOMMEMDATION...............................35

BROWN BASMATI 35

ORANGE JUICE 36

BAD FAT 37

HEALTHY FAT 37

PROTEIN 39

FAD DIETS 39

CONCLUSION 41

INTORDUCTION

YOU ARE WHAT YOU EAT

In other words, what you eat determines the condition or state of your health. Drawing from the above catch phrase, you will all agree with me that the health benefits of eating right cannot be over emphasised. Which is why in our world today natural medicine continues to gain popularity and more significance.

However, the fact still, remains that natural medicines are based on more than, a palliative approach to disease; that does not require the ingestion of patented chemicals (i.e.pharmaceuticals). Which side effects often outweigh their claimed therapeutic ones.

In spite of this, it is sad that a lot of people still prefer the ingestion of patented chemicals (pharmaceutical) as either a preventive or curative measure for staying healthy. Instead of simply managing or suppressing symptoms, through invoking bodily self-healing. In a nut shell, simply applying the strategy that removes the interference that keeps it from doing so.

In fact, in actual sense, achieving this is just a question of modifying your diet i.e – adding or eating something naturally medicinal here and removing something not so healthy there.

CHAPTER 1

MY TESTIMONY

As an African I am sharing my practical experience and not a theoretical ideology. It is what I did and I saw result. It is what I am still doing and I am still having result. I consider myself to be a health freak to an average degree, for many years but few years ago; I decided to upgrade or take my healthy lifestyle to a higher level.

Thus, I embarked on a change of diet/lifestyle without the intension of losing weight but primarily to detoxify myself. Within seven weeks I lost 10 kilos and when I suddenly lost the weight I was pleased and excited about myself both mentally and physically.

The whole drastic change brought about a new sense of an inside-outside form of transformation, which generated a great level of ecstasy that makes me feel good and great all the time. In all honesty, I am always feeling 'on top'.

I will like to draw your attention to the good thing about losing weight or maintaining a healthy lifestyle; not only will you look trim your skin will glow and you will have more energy. In other words, you become trim, more attractive, healthy, more confident and very energetic.

GLYCEMIC INDEX/ GLYCEMIC LOAD; *WHAT ARE THEY?*

As a way of laying foundation, I would like to talk about two of the crucial or key aspects, that played a major role in my new journey of staying healthy. More so, they are phrases that I will be referring to a lot in this book. These two phrases are: "Glycemic Index" and Glycemic load. To begin with, glycemic index is basically a measurement of how rapidly a particular food increases the blood sugar levels in your body. Glycemic index is relevant to food that contain some amount of carbohydrate.
So, you won't find a glycemic index chart for food items like chicken, fish and eggs.

In other words, Glycemic Index (GI) is a ranking of carbohydrate-containing food based on the overall effect on blood glucose levels. It should be noted that food that absorbed slowly have a low GI rating, while food that absorbed quickly have a higher GI rating.

Furthermore, food rich in carbohydrate are listed according to their glycemic index and they can be classified into three main categories: Low Glycemic index food, Medium glycemic index food and High glycemic index food. High glycemic index food are those that are broken down by the body very rapidly and release glucose to the body quickly. On the other hand, low glycemic index food are those that require sometime, to be broken down and the glucose is then slowly released to the body. While medium glycemic index food falls somewhere between these two categories.

HIGH GLYCEMIC

As a way of emphasis, in simple terms, high glycemic index food force the body to produce fat storing and appetite producing hormones that make you want to be eating more (insatiable). Thus, the rush of energy given by high GI food does not last and is soon followed by an energy lull. So, you get hungry and want to eat more. In a nutshell, high glycemic food makes you to have insatiable appetite.

Having this understanding at the back of one's mind, is important because choosing slowly absorbed carbohydrates, instead of quickly absorbed carbohydrates, can help even out blood glucose levels for even people suffering from diabetes.

LOW GLYCEMIC INDEX

By eating meals that have a low GI you will feel less hungry. This means that rather than controlling your cravings for food by will-power alone, you are controlling them by satisfying your body. On the low glycemic diet your desire to snack or over eat will be greatly reduced and by eating fewer calories you can easily control your weight.

HIGH GLYCEMIC AND LOW GLYCEMIC INDEX

It should be noted that, complex carbohydrates like rice, potatoes and wheat based products raise your blood sugar levels to dangerously high levels. More so, the rapid increase of blood sugar level after eating high-glycemic index food – such as white bread, potatoes, white rice, a lot of the breakfast cereal, baked food and sweets -- signals the pancreas to secrete more insulin.

Consequently, the high levels of insulin can then sharply decrease blood sugar to dangerously low levels and eventually lead to various health problems. However, eating food with a low glycemic index sustains a more even distribution of blood glucose and allows the pancreas to function more efficiently.

In addition, food is given a glycemic index score according to its effect on blood glucose levels. So, glycemic index scores are based on a scale of zero to 100, where 100 represents pure glucose. As earlier mentioned, glycemic scores are grouped into three categories low, medium and high. Food with the scores of 70 % and above is classified as high-glycemic.

Thus, food such as, white bread and white rice will have a score of 70 percent and above while

Medium-glycemic food, such as raisins, white Basmati rice, Long grain Brown rice, sweet potatoes etc will have a score of 56-69 % On the other hand, Low glycemic food such as nuts, Brown Basmati, Barley, Rye, yam, Beans, Quinoa, Oats etc will have a glycemic index of 35 – 55 %.

It should be noted that, the consumption of high-glycemic food with a value of over 70 %; over a period of time will decrease your ability to control your blood sugar levels and may lead to conditions, such as diabetes, cancer and other chronic diseases

Therefore, it is best to limit the consumption of food that has a glycemic index of over 70% because as earlier mentioned; food with a high glycemic index will make people to store belly fat, trigger hidden fires of inflammation in the body and cause fatty liver. Which can lead to the whole cascade of obesity, pre-diabetes and diabetes etc.

On the other hand, the trick and the good thing about low glycemic index food is that it makes people feel or become fuller quickly and stay longer without being hungry. In a nutshell, this explains why low glycemic food curbs hunger and suppresses appetite, which can also lead to effective weight loss and being in good health.

It is worth mentioning that, on the GI diet there is no food that you cannot eat but the secret is eating more, low GI food than high GI food. More so, low GI does not always mean low fat, so it is advisable to watch the fat content in your meals.

GLYCEMIC INDEX SCORES
Low GI   Medium GI   High GI
0-55   56-69   70 or greater

GLYCEMIC LOAD

WHAT IS GLYCEMIC LOAD?

Glycemic Load (GL) measures the portion (calories) of the food and how it raises blood sugar level. As a tool glycemic load, is more accurate compare to glycemic index (GI) because it gives a more comprehensive assessment of the impact of eating carbohydrates. In the sense that, it includes the amount of carbohydrate in a serving as well.

For instance, glycemic index value only tells how rapidly a specific carbohydrate translate into sugar. It does not tell you how much of that carbohydrate is in a serving of a specific food, which is what the glycemic load (GL) will do.

Thus, it is very important to take both the glycemic index and glycemic load into account for a better understanding of the effect of food on blood sugar. Let us look at this example, the carbohydrate in watermelon, has a high GI but there is no a lot of sugar in a serving of watermelon because most of it is fibre and water.

Consequently, watermelon's glycemic load is relatively low. In terms of the glycemic load measurement; a GL of 20 or more is considered high and a GL of 11- 19 is considered medium while a GL of 10 or less is considered low.

In addition, food that have a low GL will in most cases have a low GI while food with a medium or high GL range will in most cases have a very low to very high GI (Glycemic Load).

CAUTION

Thus, it should be noted that low GI is just one part of a healthy diet. As such, it has been suggested that, there is a tendency that you will still be eating unhealthy if you only look at the glycemic index of food without considering the glycemic load as well. For example, Peanut M&Ms have a glycemic index of 33% but that doesn't make them a healthier choice for dinner than pasta served with chili con carne, which has a GI of 40%. Instead of just looking at GI, you should look at the full scores of the glycemic load of a meal.

Thus, the overall number of the scores should be a combination of all the food you're eating together instead of each type of food on its own. Also, it has been suggested that if you are hungry within two hours of eating a meal, probably you have eaten food with a high GI—and nothing else.

As such, it is best to look for a choice of food that has a low glycemic index, mix or cooked with healthy fats plus lean sources of protein such as fish, beans, nuts and seeds for a meal. That way you will have a glycemic load that's healthy and fills you up as well.

CHAPTER 2

WHAT I DID DO FOR THE SEVEN WEEKS

For seven weeks, I stopped eating high and medium glycemic index food. Basically, I stopped eating rice of any kind and bread of any kind. In addition, I virtually stopped eating everything that was not compatible with my blood group based on the research that even if the food you are eating is healthy, if it is not compatible with your blood group, you could still have some health issues.

As a result, I stopped eating food like potatoes, cat fish, London pounded yam; I am being specific about the type of pounded yam because the original pounded is low glycemic index food which makes it a healthy option.

During this period, I was only eating skinless chicken and turkey grilled in Halogen oven with Nigerian low glycemic index food like, Moimoi and Beans. It should be noted that I only cooked the beans that was compatible with my blood group; in the different ways, we cook beans in the Nigerian culture. For instance, Ewa goyin style, beans soup (Gbegiri) etc.

Also, I continued with my habit of not eating raw sugar for many years and I replaced rice with Millet and Barley. More so, I ate Oats mixed with Barley and Pumpkin seeds as well. I snacked with Cucumber, Carrots, Almonds, Walnut and Pumpkin seeds.

In addition, I used Millet and Barley powder for tuwo, okele, fufu or swallow with okra soup, bean soup (gbegiri without palm oil) and vegetable soup (without palm oil). Also, I drank a lot of water and I ate Broccoli and flaxseed - I was drinking the flaxseed as well as drinking soaked okra in water. More so, I added salad and fruits to my diet that were compatible to my blood group and I was swimming at least twice a week.

POST SEVEN WEEKS – LIFESTYLE

Bearing in mind that, it is not only sugar that can increase blood sugar levels in the body but rather food that contain complex carbohydrates like, rice and wheat based products also raises your blood sugar levels to dangerously high levels. After my seven weeks of detoxification I began to learn how to eat carbohydrate wisely. So, as to maintain the achieved or desired result.

Consequently, I focused on the Nigerian low glycemic index food and still I am continuing with that without compromise. Example of these food are: Tuwon-shinkafa or rice fufu or okele made from Basmati rice which has the same 55 -56 % low glycemic index rate with the brown long grain rice.

I use Brown rice powder, Quinoa powder, Amala powder, Brown and White oat meal powder for my tuwo, okele, fufu or swallow. In terms of the soup to go with any of the tuwo, okele, fufu or swallow I mentioned earlier; I use either grounded Pumpkin seeds, Almonds, Sesame seeds as an alternative, to Egusi soup and I cook it with either Rapeseed oil, Olive oil, Sunflower mix with the long bell peppers; in order to give it the palm oil reddish colour effect.

However, when the Carotino Red Palm fruit and Rapeseed oil, proven to significantly lower cholesterol level came into circulation; I just switched over to that and it does give the soup that palm oil colour effect.

So, if you are someone, who is addicted to palm oil to the level that you cannot see yourself eating any soup without the red colour palm oil touch; then your 'deliverance' has come because the Carotino Red Palm Fruit and Rapeseed Oil guarantees that effect and even much more.

Also, I eat Bean soup (gbegiri), okra soup mix with ugu leaves or just by itself; ogbono soup mix with just ugu leaves or mix with okra and ugu leaves. In addition, still as part of the soup to go with the tuwo, okele, fufu or swallow: I eat Kuka soup (dried Baobab leaves) and other various African vegetable soup like spinach, bitter leave, water leaves and ugu soup, yakuwa and soborodo (Sorrel leaves), zogala leaves (moringa leaves) as well as okazi soup.

It should be noted that, as an alternative to white long grain rice I eat Brown Basmati rice and Quinoa grains. I cook both grains as Jollof, Fried rice and in all the other different ways Africans cook rice. More so, I eat both Brown and White Rice noodles and I regularly eat moi-moi and beans. In addition, I eat Acha (Digitaria exilis or Fonio or hungry rice), boiled yams and yam pottage.

Furthermore, as an alternative to the usual bread I stopped eating during my detoxification period. I mean the usual bread made from wheat (white or brown); I now eat Polish Rye bread and bread-made from grains like brown rice, or other low glycemic grains like Quinoa, Buckwheat etc.

Also, as a way of making up for all the food that can cause temptation and eventually result into going back to square one in terms of staying healthy; I created my own healthy cake recipe, meat pie and pancakes using Rye flour and Quinoa. Without using the conventional flour made from wheat. Still I only eat skinless chicken and turkey meat. Plus, fish with low saturated fat like; Mackerel, Sardines, Salmon, Tilapia, Stock fish etc and other sea food: like prawns, snails, shrimps, squid and less quantity of mussels because of the little bit of the saturated fat in them. In addition, I sometimes use Palm Fruit and Rapeseed oil to make Akra. (Bean cake).

It should be noted that I still eat my salad and fruits specifically fruits with low sugar content like pear, plums etc. Also, I only drink sugar free Almond and Soya milk and I eat sugar free Almond or Soya yoghurt. In addition, I snack with fruits like Black Velvet Tamarind and Baobab fruit; it should be noted that not only can these two fruits be enjoyed as smoothie but they are full of excellent health benefits which include regulating blood sugar levels as well as maintaining a healthy blood pressure.

Also, I eat Pomegranate fruits and beside snacking with Brown rice cakes, Quinoa cakes, Buckwheat cakes and sugar free biscuits and drinks. I also, snack with homemade Quinoa and Rye bread cake with Walnut and Pumpkin seeds as well as Rye and Brown rice bread cake with other nuts and seeds.

More so, as a pattern I eat some other food simply by checking the calories, sugar content, saturated percentage of the fat to ensure they are very low and high in poly-saturated and mono-unsaturated before I consume them.

Also, I eat nuts and seeds that contain good fat which lowers LDL cholesterol (bad cholesterol) and increase HDL cholesterol (Good one); like Almonds, Walnuts, Sesame seeds, Pumpkin seed etc. More so, any time I fancy eating butter, I eat Soya butter, Almond butter, Tahini (Sasame butter) as well as Benecol and Pro- active butter which has been proven to lower cholesterol.

You could be wondering in your mind; wait a minute! 'How on earth is this woman coping with not eating food and snacks or drinks she has been used to since she was a child?' Well, the shocking good news is that I am not missing out of the type of food I have always been used to! All I am doing now is eating the healthy version of my cultural cuisine and you can do the same.

My pattern of healthy lifestyle is easier to follow than being restricted on a specific diet and pattern of consuming the food per se because you can eat just like you would normally do; for instance, your three-square meals and you do not have to worry about dividing the food into portions like it has been advocated for, for many years.

In as much as it is a great and effective strategy if one is discipline enough to adhere to it. However, the down side is, the tenacity and the ability to maintain it for a long period of time, especially the days you get so hungry that you cannot control your hunger, for one reason or the other without falling back to square.

On the other hand, with the low glycemic index food you cannot eat too much because it fills you up quickly. Hence, the reason why dividing the food into portion is not a requirement because you cannot eat more than a certain portion, except you want to throw up and you do not get hungry for a long time.

For example, you will notice that no matter how hungry you are the portion of beans that will fill you up is less compare to the portion of white long grain rice you will normally consume and this is just because beans is a low glycemic index food.

It should be noted that, for any healthy lifestyle to be complete, authentic and effective physical exercise must be part and parcel of it. So, as a form of physical exercise, I go swimming, I walk a lot, I do some rigorous jumping in the house, I Dance and I play Badminton when I have the opportunity.

CHAPTER 3

SPECIFIC FOOD RECOMMENDATION

- Eat okra because it is very healthy and medicinal. According to research,

- I recommend spinach, Ugu, Okazi, Cassava leaves, Ewedu, Potato leaves and all the other green vegetables we eat in Africa.

- Bell peppers, red and white onions, spring onions and garlic are healthy and medicinal because they have antibiotic elements.

- Sweet Potato can be eaten because it is gluten free and has a medium glycemic index.

- Although white potato is medium glycemic but the gluten in it stores fat round the waist which is why it is not a good healthy option.

- Eat boiled yam, yam pottage (Asaro or paten doya) cooked without sugar and the real pounded yam. Also, eat Amala.

- Cassava is full of protein than carbohydrate which makes it a healthy option when it's cooked and eaten with other healthy ingredients and food.

- Quinoa, Brown Basmati, Barley, Millet and sorghum can be eaten as a replacement for rice or couscous and the powder can be used for tuwo or okele or swallow for the Nigerians and for the Ghanians and other African countries fufu.

- Wholegrain or non-wholegrain Oats powder can also be used for tuwo, Okele, swallow or fufu or as porridge.

- Although, green plantain fufu is low glycemic. However, I am skeptical about recommending it because the research on eating according to your blood group; suggests that plantain is not good for any blood group

- You can eat corn as well if it is compatible with your blood group.

- Beans can be eaten alone, or in the form of moi moi or Soup (Gbegiri) or even mix with other grains.

- Sorrel (yakuwa and soborodo) can be eaten in various ways.

- Acha can be eaten (Digitaria exilis, Fonio or hungry rice) as porridge (kunu or ogi) soup, pate (pottage), tuwo, Okele or fufu.

- Sorghum (Dawa or guinea corn) can be used for tuwo or okele or fufu or even porridge (ogi or kunu)

- Use grounded Pumpkin seeds, Almonds, sesame seeds as egusi alternative. For all your cooking use either Rapeseed oil, Olive oil, Sunflower oil mix with the long bell peppers. So, your soup will look like the soup that has been cooked with Palm oil or just use Carotino Red Palm fruit and Rapeseed oil alone.

- Based on research, Ogbono (African wild Mango Seed) lowers cholesterol and aids weidght loss. So, Ogbono cooked with ugu leaves or your favourite vegetable is another healthy option to go with your tuwo, Okele. Or fufu.

- Eat Kuka soup (dried Baobab leaves) and other various African vegetable soup like spinach, bitter leaves, ugu leaves, water leaves, Yakuwa and Soborodo leaves (Sorrel leaves), zogala leaves (moringa leaves) as well as okazi leaves.

- For lovers of Masa/Waina, a type of delicacy eaten in the Northern part of Nigeria; you can also use brown Basmati rice, Millet, Barley or Sorghum (dawa) for Masa as long you use healthy cooking oil like rapeseed oil, Olive oil, Carotino red palm fruit and rapeseed oil etc.

- You can use Palm fruit and Rapeseed oil to make akara (Bean cake)

- Eat low GI whole grain and non-wholegrain bread like Rye Bread, Ezekiel Bread, Rice Bread e.tc

- Also, eat food such as Rice Noodles and Buckwheat.

- **REMOVE** all of these from your diet: Nigerian Big Mama Bread, Agege Bread etc, Hard dough bread, wheat white and brown Bread, Long grain white rice, London potato and Farina Pounded yam, Nigerian fufu (Akpu) and Ghanian Kenkey.

- **REMOVE** raw sugar of any kind from your diet.

SNACKING HABIT WILL NOT SUFFER

Snacking habit addiction? Don't worry you are not alone! There are varieties of healthy snacks that will satisfy your cravings; so, relax and enjoy the following snacks at your disposal: Quinoa chips, 'by Eat Real', Various brands of Brown rice cakes lightly salted; carrots, cucumber, fruits especially the ones with less sugar contents like certain apples, plums, pear etc.

In addition, nuts/seeds like almonds, walnuts, flaxseeds, pumpkin seeds, sesame seeds etc. Also, sweet potato chips; orange, purple and white sweet potato chips by 'Scott Farms' and other brands. Ryvita flatbread, crisp bread and crackers especially mix grains and Jacobs brand as well.

WHY I HAD TO STOP THE WHEAT PRODUCTS

Research has shown that due to the process of genetically modifying food like wheat etc the present- day wheat unlike the olden days is not good for any anyone because the gluten in the wheat makes people to blow up and the gluten stores fat around the waist line just like the gluten in white potatoes.

For a broader understanding, it is not only the wheat products and the gluten in white potatoes that store fat around your waistline but research has also shown that cartoon juice; like orange juice and apple juice etc are not healthy as well because both the sugar contents and other additives store fat around the waist line when consumed.

Thus, nothing can substitute freshly, squeezed, homemade juice. However, water is still the healthiest of all and nothing can beat that.

According to research, the biggest problem is wheat and the major source of gluten in our diet. Having said that, the gluten in the wheat is not just the problem. There are other hidden components responsible for weight gain, obesity and diseases such as, diabetes, heart disease, cancer, dementia and more.

Sadly, this tsunami of chronic illnesses is on the increase because a vast majority of people are still consuming our beloved diet staple; wheat bread and all the other wheat products hidden in everything from soups, lipsticks to envelope adhesive.

To narrow it down to the African community, in the same vein, majority of Africans consume a large amount of wheat flour every year through eating, African type of bread, meat pie, wheat fufu or tuwo, puff – puff, cakes and pastries.

It should be noted that according to research, the reason our modern wheat is the biggest problem; is because it contains a super starch called amylopectin A which is super fattening. Also, it contains a form of super gluten and it is equally super-inflammatory. More so, it contains forms of a super drug that is super-addictive and makes you to crave and want to eat more.

Thus, drawing from these components of our modern wheat there is no difference between the whole wheat and white flour. Which explains the argument that, now two slices of whole wheat bread can raise your blood sugar more than two tablespoons of table sugar.

CHAPTER 4

WHY I CHOSE SOME OF THE LOW GLYCEMIC INDEX FOOD I EAT NOW

BENEFITS OF YAMS

According to research, yams contain relatively little protein and in a 1-cup serving of yams which is nearly 40 grams almost all the carbohydrates are healthy complex carbs. Also, yams are rich in fiber, a type of carbohydrate your body does not digest.

Although, fiber is not a source of energy however, it helps in maintaining a healthy digestive tract and it is associated with a decreased risk of heart disease, obesity and some forms of cancer. More so, due to the fact, that **yams contain more fibre and less sugar, as such it does not raise your blood sugar levels.**

In addition, another good news for lovers of yams is that they are extremely low in fat and contributes less than 0.25 grams per 1-cup of serving. In as much as dietary fat is essential for maintaining healthy cell membranes.

However, loading your organs and allowing your body to absorb fat-soluble vitamins- too much dietary fat, can lead to cardiovascular disease. Implicitly the low-fat content of yams is able, to reduce your overall dietary fat consumption to a healthy level.

Furthermore, yams are an excellent source of vitamins C and B6 and 1 cup of serving provides approximately 20 percent of your daily requirement of each of these nutrients. More so, yams have a lot of Manganese, copper and potassium which are essential minerals and 1-cup of serving provides roughly about 20 percent of each of these essential minerals.

Thus, drawing from the above -mentioned benefits of yams, it is evident that eating the original Pounded yam made from yams and Amala which is also made from yams with the right soup; yam pottage without added sugar or palm oil and boiled yams with the right stew or accomplishment; are indeed some of the African cuisine healthy options that Africans can continue to enjoy. Hurray!

BENEFITS OF OATMEAL

Based on research findings, Oatmeal can help you to lose weight because it increases the production of the satiety hormone responsible for making individuals not to be hungry for a long period of time.

Also, because it contains the soluble fiber beta-glucan it improves insulin sensitivity and helps to lower blood sugar levels. In addition, due to the content of a powerful antioxidant, avenanthramides in Oatmeal; Oatmeal lowers the risk of heart disease by reducing the LDL cholesterol as well as lowering your blood pressure. More so, oats are very high in many vitamins and minerals.

BENEFITS OF QUINOA

Quinoa has twice protein content compare to Barley or Rice. Also, it is among the least allergenic of all the grains and that makes it a fantastic wheat-free choice. Beside the fact that quinoa contains a good level of several vitamins like Vitamin B and E.

It is high in anti-inflammatory phytonutrients which makes it potentially beneficial for prevention and treatment of disease. In addition, research has also, shown that Quinoa aids weight loss due to its high insoluble fiber and protein.

BENEFITS OF RYE

Like other low glycemic index food the benefits of rye include a decreased risk of diabetes, cardiovascular disease, diverticulitis, constipation, gallstones and cancer, decreased inflammation, insulin-resistance and LDL cholesterol and it does aid weight loss – it flattens the stomach.

BENEFITS OF BUCKWHEAT

According to research Buckwheat improves the health of the heart by lowering cholesterol and blood pressure levels. Also, it contains disease-fighting antioxidants and provides highly digestible protein.

In addition, due to its high content of fibre it helps to improve digestion as well as prevent Diabetes. More so, it is gluten free, non-allergenic and does contain important Vitamins and Minerals.

CHAPTER 5

GENERAL RECOMMEMDATION

BROWN BASMATI

Many people are under the false notion that only sugars can increase blood sugar levels in the body. However, we now know it is not so because food that contain complex carbohydrates like rice, potatoes and wheat based products also raises your blood sugar levels to dangerously high levels. So, in terms of the best rice to eat, although Basmati rice is a medium glycemic index food. However, Brown Basmati rice has a considerably low glycemic index than white Basmati rice.

As such, it does make a lot of sense to consume more of Brown Basmati rice especially those aspiring to become health freaks like myself or those suffering from chronic diseases. It should be noted that, other types of rice like long grain rice, short grain sticky rice and risotto rice have a high glycemic index and should be avoided by people who are trying to battle their bulge or what to stay healthy.

As mentioned earlier, people who are suffering from either chronic diseases or are trying to lose weight or stay healthy should always eat low or medium glycemic index food. This will help them to regulate their blood sugar levels more so, lead to greater satiety. High glycemic index food restores or gives energy quickly when the blood sugar level increases but within a short time the blood sugar level will crash and make the person hungrier which will eventually lead to overeating.

Considering the fact, that nutritionally rice is mostly starch and doesn't add a whole lot of nutrients to our meals other than carbohydrate. Thus, consuming your rice meal with protein food and vegetables will add nutrients and lower the overall GI of the meal. In addition, dishes you previously use rice to make, can be nutritionally enhanced by swapping with other forms of more nutritious grains such as barley and quinoa etc.

ORANGE JUICE

As earlier mentioned, the worst thing you can do to your body is to start the day with a glass of orange juice which is contrary to the belief that people have held unto for years; that it is the best way to start your day. It should be noted that most concentrated juices like; cranberry juice, Apple and grape juice etc cause more problem around your waistline. This is due to, the fact that they contain more sugar than some of the fizzy drinks.

More so, during the process of making the concentrated juice the fibre content, gets lost and in actual sense, it is the fibre that helps, in burning the fat. In other words, it aids weight loss. Thus, endeavour to eat fruits and vegetables for their high vitamin and mineral content. Try to eat plenty of fresh fruit and vegetables, rather than canned ones that often contain added sugar or salt.

BAD FAT

Cut off bad fat in your diet and unhealthy fats include both trans fats and saturated fats. These fats will raise your LDL cholesterol and elevated LDL cholesterol is associated with heart disease. Food high in trans fats include food made with partially hydrogenated oils," such as butter or margarine. Baked food, fried food like chicken and chips, Puff-puff, Akara fried with hydrogenated oil or saturated fat oil etc.

Frozen pizza, and other highly processed food often contain trans fats. Examples of food high in saturated fats are: pizza, cheese, red meat, and full-fat dairy products. Coconut oil is also high in saturated fat but it can also increase good cholesterol.

HEALTHY FAT

It is wise to eat healthy fats in moderation. By saying healthy fat, I mean poly-unsaturated, mono-unsaturated and omega-3 fats which are all good lifestyle choices. These good fats lower your LDL cholesterol and raise your HDL cholesterol. Good oils include Olive oil, Canola oil, Soya, Almond oil, Sunflower oil, Sesame oil, Rapeseed oil and Red palm fruit mixed with Rapeseed oil.

More so, swap the unhealthy butter with butter like; Soya butter, Almond butter and Tahini with low salt or without salt (Sesame seed butter), Pro-active and Benecol. Both Pro- active and Benecol have been proven to lower your cholesterol.

Fish are high in omega-3 fatty acids especially salmon, tuna, trout, mackerel, sardines, squid, mussels, herring etc. Plant sources like flaxseed, plant oils, nuts and seeds are also good source of healthy fat. Although your body doesn't process the fats from these as effectively. However, like I mentioned earlier on it is best to eat healthy fat in moderation.

CARB

Remove White or Brown wheat bread, Long grain White rice and Potatoes from your diet. Instead eat Sweet Potatoes, Cassava, other grains and seeds such as Long grain Brown rice, Basmati Rice, Brown Basmati rice, white or Brown Rice Noodles, Buckwheat and Quinoa.

Do not eat raw sugar of any kind but eat a variety of whole food (with low GI) instead of processed food because whole food offers a balance of healthy carbohydrates and do not forget to only eat low GI bread like; Rye Bread Ezekiel Bread, Rice Bread, Quinoa Bread, Buckwheat bread etc.

.

PROTEIN

Choose white meat; like skinless Chicken/ Turkey, lean meat, beans and tofu for their protein content. Also, include healthy fish and sea food mentioned previously. More so, inculcate the habit of eating low-fat dairy products like: Skimmed milk, reduced fat cheeses and non- dairy products like: Soya Milk, Almond Milk and Rice Milk because they will reduce your fat intake while ensuring that you receive enough calcium.

Make physical activities like Walking, Dancing, going to the Gym, Swimming etc part and parcel of your lifestyle because it enhances healthy lifestyle.

FAD DIETS

Stay away from fad diets; like liquid diets, diet pills and other diet supplements unless you are under the supervision of a physician. It should be noted that research has shown that liquid diets can result into Dehydration, electrolyte imbalance which can damage the liver.

Generally, if a diet plan or product does any of the following:

•   Promises extremely quick weight loss (more than 1-2 pounds per week),
•   Promises to help you lose weight without changing your habits.
•   Requires you to spend a lot of money.
•   Restricts your food choices and doesn't encourage balanced nutrition.

Be warned! it's probably a fad.

Lastly, avoid yo-yo healthy lifestyle. Once you have lost the weight or detoxified your self be grateful for your improved lifestyle; then work hard to maintain your weight or stay healthy instead of cycling up and down the scale.

CONCLUSION

Remember as I mentioned earlier; high glycemic index food force the body to produce fat storing and appetite producing hormones that make you want to be eating more. In other words, it makes you to have insatiable appetite.

Thus, it affects your weight, waste line and for some it affects even their self – esteem and increases the risk of serious illnesses or diseases. So, I believe it is worth swapping the high glycemic index food with the low glycemic index food. Interestingly, with the low glycemic healthy lifestyle, you will discover that you do not have to indulge in a kind of a super- perfect diet to begin to see encouraging progress in a matter of days.

All you need, to lose weight and stay healthy is already packed in the African food. You only need to really know what eating and staying healthy means because it is not what most people think it is. I know we are so wrapped up with the belief system or culture of inculcating the habit of going to the gym or engaging in one form of exercise or the other; although there are health benefits of doing all of that.

However, I will like to submit to you that you cannot exercise your way out with a poor or wrong diet.

Thus, losing weight or detoxifying oneself or even staying healthy is not about eating carrots, celery or cucumber. It is about eating the right carb with the right amount of protein and the fat will just burn off naturally. It is that simple!

As my last nugget and way of emphasis, a healthy lifestyle leaves you fit, energetic and lowers the risk of any chronic disease.

Finally, I challenge you to rise-up now! Pick up from wherever you are and embark on this great, rewarding, highly beneficial and fulfilling journey of a change of lifestyle! I promise! You will be glad you did! All it takes is the discipline and if God did it for me; I am confident he will help you as well. Just be determine and God will help you to finish the rest.

Be rest assured that if I can do it, you can do it! So, go for it! Just remember to do what I did! Plug into the power source; ask God for the grace to go on this great journey and he will give it to you like he did for me. See you at the top!

REFERENCES

www.livestrong.com

PATIENT HANDOUT 4 University of Wisconsin Integrative Medicine www.fammed.wisc.edu/integrative

The "New" Glucose Revolution by Jennie BrandMiller, Thomas M.S. Wolever, Stephen Colagiuri and Kaye Foster-Powell and the website www.mendosa.com/gilists.htm

http://www.glycemicindex.com/ (University of Sydney's Website)

http://diabetes.about.com/library/mendosagi/ngilists .htm

http://www.health.harvard.edu/newsweek/Glycemic _index_and_glycemic_load_for_100_foods.htm

[i] Parvin Mirmiran, Zahra Bahadoran, Mahdieh Golzarand, Asadolah Rajab, Fereidoun Azizi. **Ardeh (Sesamum indicum) Could Improve Serum Triglycerides and Atherogenic Lipid Parameters in Type 2 Diabetic Patients: A Randomized Clinical Trial. Eur J Prev Cardiol.** 2013 Apr;20(2):202-8. doi: 10.1177/2047487312437625. Epub 2012 Jan 25.

[ii] Kalliopi Karatzi, Kimon Stamatelopoulos, Maritta Lykka, Pigi Mantzouratou, Sofia Skalidi, Nikolaos Zakopoulos, Christos Papamichael, Labros S Sidossis. Sesame oil consumption exerts a beneficial effect on endothelial function in hypertensive men. Eur J Prev Cardiol. 2012 Jan 25. Epub 2012 Jan 25. PMID: 22345690

[iii] Devarajan Sankar, Amanat Ali, Ganapathy Sambandam, Ramakrishna Rao. Sesame oil exhibits synergistic effect with anti-diabetic medication in patients with type 2 diabetes mellitus. Clin Nutr. 2011 Jun ;30(3):351-8. Epub 2010 Dec 16. PMID: 21163558

[iv] D Sankar, M Ramakrishna Rao, G Sambandam, K V Pugalendi. A pilot study of open label sesame oil in hypertensive diabetics. J Med Food. 2006 Fall;9(3):408-12. PMID: 17004907